What is a doula?
The Guidebook for Every Family

By: La'Joi Carter

Preface

Welcome to "What is a Doula? The Guidebook for Every Family," a comprehensive resource designed to demystify the role of doulas in the birthing process and beyond. This book is born out of a passion for supporting families during one of the most transformative periods of their lives—pregnancy, birth, and the postpartum journey. Whether you are expecting your first child, exploring options for additional support during birth, or simply curious about the role of doulas in modern maternity care, this guide is for you.

The concept of a doula, a professional trained to provide emotional, physical, and educational support to a birthing person and their family, is ancient but has seen a resurgence in recent years as more families seek personalized and compassionate care. Doulas serve as advocates, educators, and comforting presences, offering a continuum of care that is often missing in traditional healthcare settings.

Our journey through these pages will take you from the historical roots of doula care to the practicalities of finding and working with a doula that fits your family's unique needs. We'll explore the different types of doulas, the evidence-based benefits of doula support, and how to navigate the process of integrating a doula into your birth team. Our goal is not only to inform but also to empower you and your family to make choices that align with your values, preferences, and circumstances.

This book is a collaborative effort, drawing on the wisdom and experiences of doulas, healthcare professionals, and families who have walked this path before you. Through their stories and insights, I aim to provide a well-rounded perspective on what it means to have a doula by your side.

As you turn these pages, I hope to inspire confidence, provide comfort, and foster a deeper understanding of the invaluable role doulas play in the birthing community. May this guidebook serve as a beacon of light for you and your family, illuminating the path to a supported, empowered, and memorable birthing experience.

Welcome to the beginning of a beautiful journey.

Sincerely,

La'Joi Carter

Introduction

The birth of a child is a profound and deeply personal experience, one that is as old as humanity itself yet uniquely individual in its unfolding. In recent decades, the landscape of childbirth and postpartum care has shifted dramatically, with an increasing emphasis on personalized, supportive, and holistic care. Amidst these changes, one role has emerged to the forefront as a beacon of support, advocacy, and guidance: the doula.

But what exactly is a doula? This question, while seemingly straightforward, opens the door to a world of nuanced care, ancient traditions, and modern practices that support families through pregnancy, childbirth, and the postnatal period. A doula is more than just a support person; they are educators, coaches, advocates, and confidants, playing a crucial role in enhancing the birthing experience and supporting the family through one of life's most significant transitions.

This book, "What is a Doula? The Guidebook for Every Family," is designed to explore the multifaceted role of doulas and the incredible impact they can have on birth outcomes, family bonding, and the overall well-being of parents and children. Our mission is to provide you with a comprehensive understanding of what doulas do, how they fit into the broader picture of maternity care, and why they might be a valuable addition to your birthing journey.

Throughout this guide, we will delve into the historical roots of doula care, highlighting how this ancient practice has evolved to meet the needs of modern families. We'll explore the different types of doulas—birth doulas, postpartum doulas, bereavement doulas, and more—each specializing in supporting families through specific aspects of the childbearing year. We'll examine the evidence-based benefits of doula support, from reduced intervention rates and shorter labor to improved satisfaction with the birth experience and stronger parent-infant bonding.

Choosing to invite a doula into your birthing journey is a deeply personal decision, one that may raise questions and considerations unique to your situation. This guide is here to answer those questions, offering insights into how to find and choose the right doula for your family, what to expect when working with a doula, and how to make the most of this partnership.

Whether you are a first-time parent navigating the unknown waters of childbirth, a seasoned parent seeking a different experience for your next birth, or simply curious about the role of doulas in contemporary maternity care, this book is for you. Our aim is to empower you with knowledge, inspire you with stories of strength and support, and guide you toward making

informed choices that resonate with your personal beliefs,

values, and circumstances.

Let us embark on this journey together, exploring the ancient

wisdom and modern practice of doula care, and discover how a

doula can enhance and transform the birth experience for every

family.

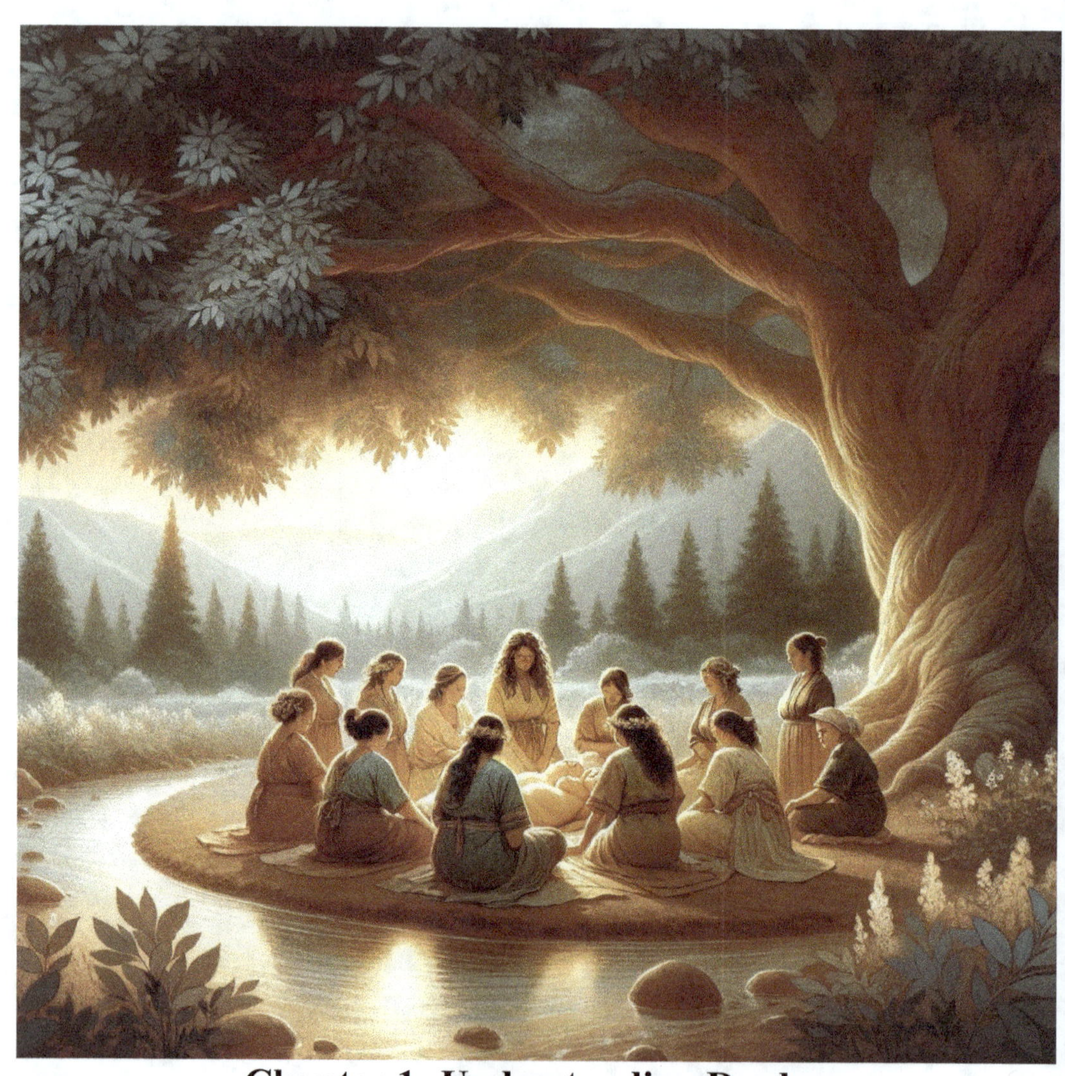

Chapter 1: Understanding Doulas

The Essence of Doula Care

At the heart of doula care is a simple yet profound commitment: to provide continuous, personalized support to families during one of life's most significant transitions. The word "doula" derives from ancient Greek, meaning "a woman who serves." Today, this role has expanded beyond its original definition to encompass a professional support person trained and experienced in childbirth and the postpartum period, offering non-medical, emotional, physical, and informational support to the birthing person and their family.

The Historical Roots of Doula Care

The practice of women supporting women through childbirth is as old as humanity itself. Throughout history and across cultures, birthing individuals have been surrounded by a community of women providing knowledge, comfort, and encouragement. This communal birthing practice ensured that the wisdom of childbirth was passed down through generations, emphasizing the natural and communal aspects of birth.

In the late 20th century, as childbirth moved from home to hospital settings in many parts of the world, the intimate, personalized support historically provided by these communities began to diminish. It was within this context that the modern doula role emerged, inspired by the desire to reintegrate continuous, supportive care into the childbirth experience, regardless of the setting.

Types of Doulas

The doula profession has diversified to meet varying family needs and preferences. While all doulas are united by their foundational commitment to support, there are several specialized roles within the field:

- **Birth Doula**: Supports families through the prenatal period, labor, and birth. They offer emotional support, physical comfort measures, and informational resources to help families make informed decisions about their birthing experience.

- **Postpartum Doula**: Provides support to the family in the first weeks or months following the birth. Their focus is on helping with newborn care, offering breastfeeding support, and assisting with household tasks to facilitate a smooth transition for the family.

- **Bereavement Doula**: Specializes in supporting families through loss, such as miscarriage, stillbirth, or infant death. They provide emotional support, guidance, and resources to help families navigate their grief.

- **Full-Spectrum Doula**: Offers support across all reproductive experiences, including birth, postpartum, miscarriage, abortion, and fertility challenges, recognizing the wide spectrum of reproductive health experiences.

The Role of a Doula

Doulas provide support tailored to the family's needs, wishes, and circumstances. They work alongside medical professionals, complementing medical care with emotional, physical, and informational support. It's important to note that doulas do not perform medical tasks or make decisions for the family. Instead, they empower families to make informed choices and advocate for their own needs and preferences.

Emotional Support: Doulas offer continuous reassurance, encouragement, and comfort. They help families navigate the emotional highs and lows of the childbearing process, fostering a sense of confidence and calm.

Physical Support: Through techniques such as massage, positioning, and breathing strategies, doulas help manage labor discomfort and support the physiological process of childbirth.

Informational Support: Doulas provide evidence-based information and resources, helping families make informed decisions about their care. They clarify medical jargon and procedures, ensuring families understand their options.

The Evolution of Doula Care

As awareness of the benefits of doula support grows, so does the demand for these services. The doula profession continues to evolve, with increasing recognition within the healthcare system and expanding access through insurance coverage and hospital-based programs. This evolution reflects a broader shift towards more personalized, respectful, and holistic maternity care.

Understanding the role and history of doulas is the first step in appreciating the depth and value they bring to the childbirth experience. As we delve deeper into the world of doula care, it becomes clear that doulas are more than just support persons; they are vital advocates for the birthing person's well-being, autonomy, and empowerment. Through their dedicated presence, doulas weave a thread of continuity and care through the tapestry of childbirth, enriching the experience for the entire family.

In the following chapters, we will explore the benefits of doula support, how to choose the right doula for your family, and how to work effectively with your doula to achieve a positive birthing experience.

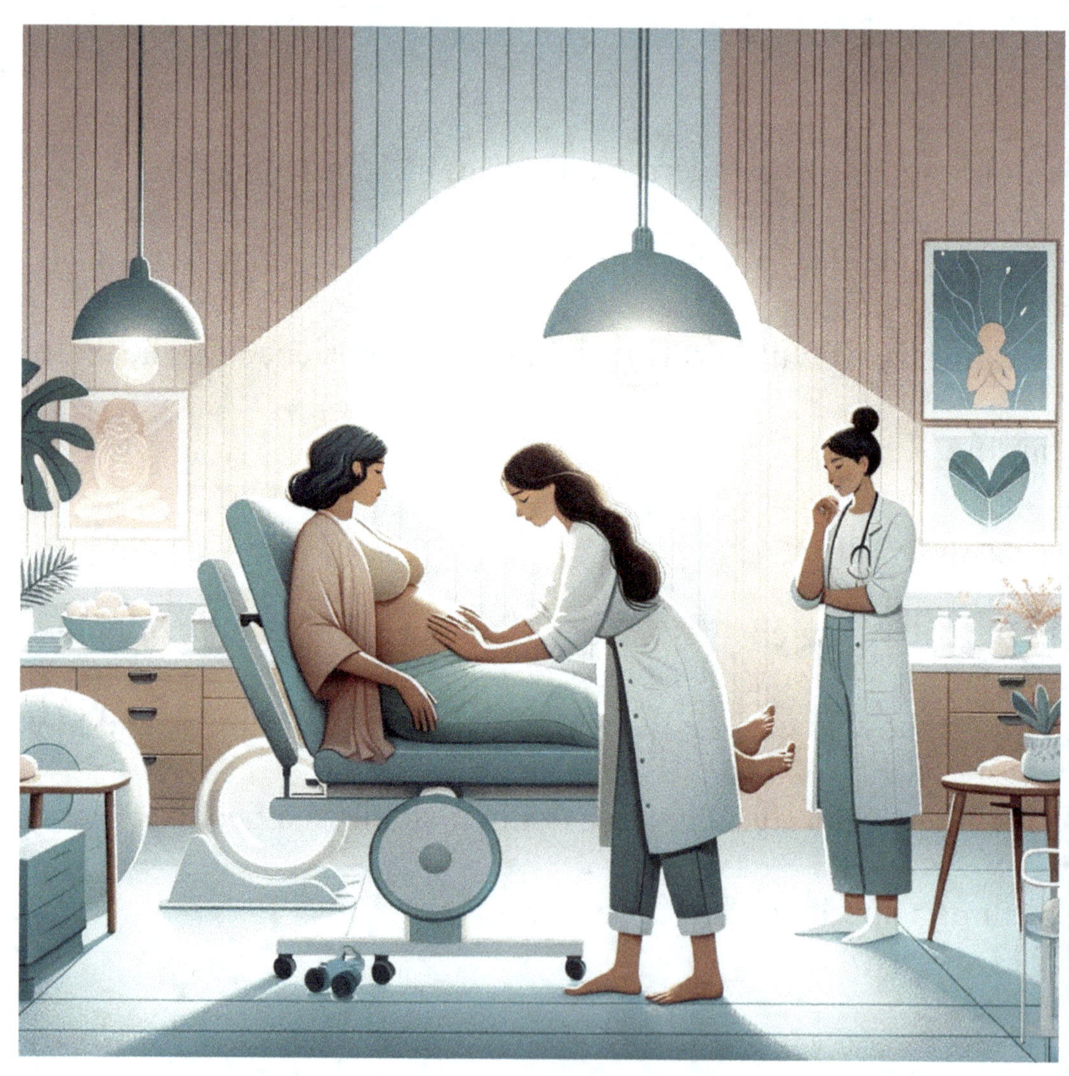

Chapter 2: The Role of a Doula

In exploring the multifaceted role of a doula, it's essential to understand the depth and breadth of support they provide to families during pregnancy, birth, and the postpartum period. Doulas are not just present at the moment of birth; their support encompasses the entire journey, from the first trimester to the weeks following the baby's arrival. This chapter delves into how doulas support families through each of these critical stages, offering a blend of emotional, physical, and informational support tailored to each family's unique needs.

During Pregnancy

Building a Relationship: The foundation of doula support begins long before labor starts. Doulas meet with families during pregnancy to build a trusting relationship, understand their preferences and fears, and discuss their birth plan. This relationship-building is crucial for establishing a comfort level that allows the birthing person to be vulnerable and empowered during labor and birth.

Educational Support: Doulas provide families with evidence-based information on pregnancy, childbirth, and newborn care. They help families navigate their options for birth settings, pain management, and interventions, ensuring that decisions are informed and aligned with the family's values and desires.

Preparation for Birth: Through prenatal visits, doulas offer guidance on preparing physically and emotionally for childbirth. They may suggest exercises for optimal fetal positioning, techniques for labor management, and strategies for effective communication with healthcare providers.

During Labor and Birth

Emotional Presence: Doulas provide continuous emotional support throughout labor and birth, offering encouragement and reassurance. Their presence helps reduce anxiety and fear, contributing to a more positive birth experience.

Physical Comfort: Doulas are skilled in non-medical pain relief techniques, such as massage, counterpressure, breathing techniques, and position changes. They assist in creating a comfortable environment, whether at home, in a birth center, or a hospital, adapting to the needs of the birthing person.

Advocacy and Information: Doulas help families communicate with healthcare providers, ensuring that their birth plan is respected and that they have the information needed to make informed decisions. They provide clarity on medical procedures and potential interventions, empowering families to advocate for their preferences.

Postpartum Support

Initial Adjustments: In the first hours and days after birth, doulas assist with the initial adjustments to parenthood, including breastfeeding support, newborn care, and emotional processing of the birth experience.

Ongoing Support: Postpartum doulas offer extended support at home, helping with infant care, meal preparation, and light household tasks. They provide a listening ear for new parents navigating the emotional and physical changes post-birth, offering guidance on infant feeding, sleep strategies, and self-care for the birthing person.

Resource Connection: Doulas connect families with community resources for further support, such as lactation consultants, parent groups, and mental health professionals specializing in postpartum care.

The role of a doula encompasses far more than the physical presence during childbirth. Doulas are a source of comfort, knowledge, and advocacy, supporting families through the transformational journey of bringing a new life into the world. They adapt their approach to meet the unique needs of each family, offering personalized care that complements the medical care provided by healthcare professionals. Through their dedicated support, doulas help families experience birth as a positive, empowering event, laying a strong foundation for the journey into parenthood.

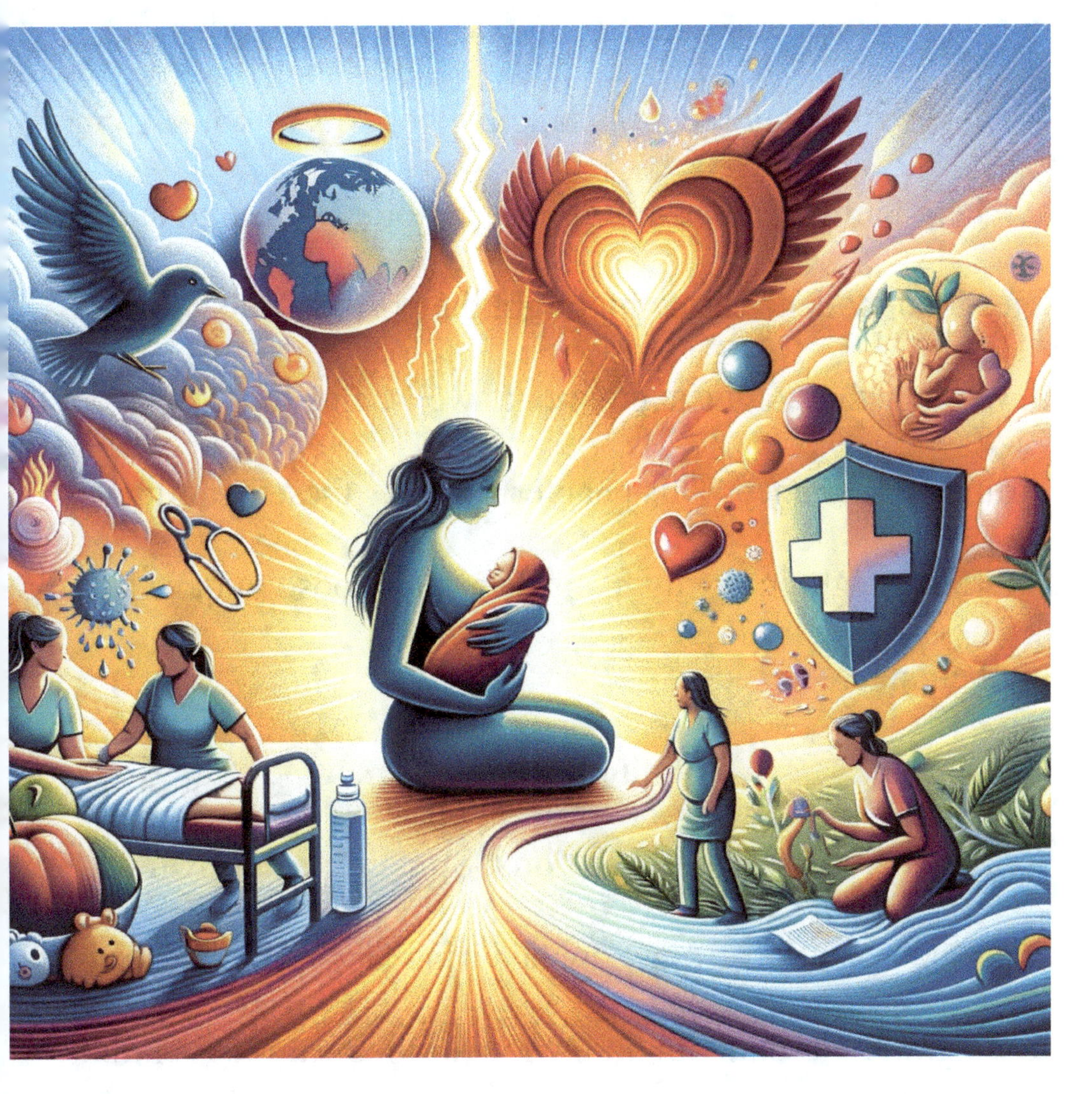

Chapter 3: Benefits of Having a Doula

The decision to involve a doula in the childbirth process is deeply personal and varies from one family to another. However, understanding the tangible benefits of doula support can help families make an informed choice. Research and anecdotal evidence alike highlight the positive impact doulas have on birth outcomes, emotional well-being, and the overall birthing experience. This chapter explores these benefits, offering insight into why many families choose to have a doula by their side.

For the Birthing Person

Reduced Need for Interventions: Studies have shown that continuous support from a doula during labor and birth can lead to a significant reduction in the rate of medical interventions, including cesarean sections, the use of vacuum or forceps, and the need for pitocin to induce labor. Doulas support the physiological process of birth through non-medical means, promoting a smoother and often quicker labor.

Pain Management: With a doula's guidance on breathing techniques, labor positions, and comfort measures, many birthing persons report more effective management of labor pain. This support can lead to a decreased need for pharmacological pain relief, including epidurals, allowing for a more alert and engaged birth experience.

Emotional Well-being: The emotional support provided by a doula before, during, and after birth plays a crucial role in the birthing person's mental health. Doulas offer a comforting presence, reduce anxiety and fear, and can help mitigate the risk of postpartum depression by ensuring the birthing person feels supported, heard, and empowered.

For the Partner and Family

Enhanced Involvement: Partners often feel more involved and useful in the birth process when a doula is present. Doulas can guide partners in how best to support the birthing person, fostering a collaborative and supportive environment. This guidance helps partners experience the birth as a shared, positive event.

Stress Reduction: Knowing a professional support person is present can significantly reduce stress for both the birthing person and their partner. Partners, in particular, may find comfort in having a doula to rely on for informational support and to share the emotional and physical workload.

Family Dynamics: Doulas understand the importance of integrating the entire family into the birth experience as desired. They can facilitate bonding moments immediately after birth and offer guidance on sibling integration, helping to strengthen family connections during this transformative time.

Evidence-Based Benefits

A significant body of research underscores the benefits of doula support:

- **Improved Birth Outcomes**: The presence of a doula is associated with shorter labors, fewer complications, and lower rates of intervention. Families working with doulas report higher satisfaction with their birth experiences.

- **Increased Success in Breastfeeding:** Immediate and knowledgeable support post-birth has been shown to improve breastfeeding outcomes. Doulas provide encouragement, positioning help, and latch assessment, contributing to successful breastfeeding initiation.

- **Greater Maternal Satisfaction**: Birthing persons who have the support of a doula often feel more satisfied with their birth experience, feeling a greater sense of achievement and empowerment.

The benefits of having a doula support during pregnancy, birth, and the postpartum period extend far beyond the delivery room. Doulas contribute to a more positive, empowered, and satisfying birth experience for the entire family. They provide invaluable physical, emotional, and informational support that complements the medical care received from healthcare providers, filling a critical gap in the maternity care system.

By fostering a supportive, informed, and comforting environment, doulas play a pivotal role in helping families navigate the challenges and joys of childbirth. As research continues to affirm the benefits of doula care, more families are choosing to include doulas in their birth teams, recognizing their unique ability to transform the birth experience into one of

empowerment, joy, and profound bonding.

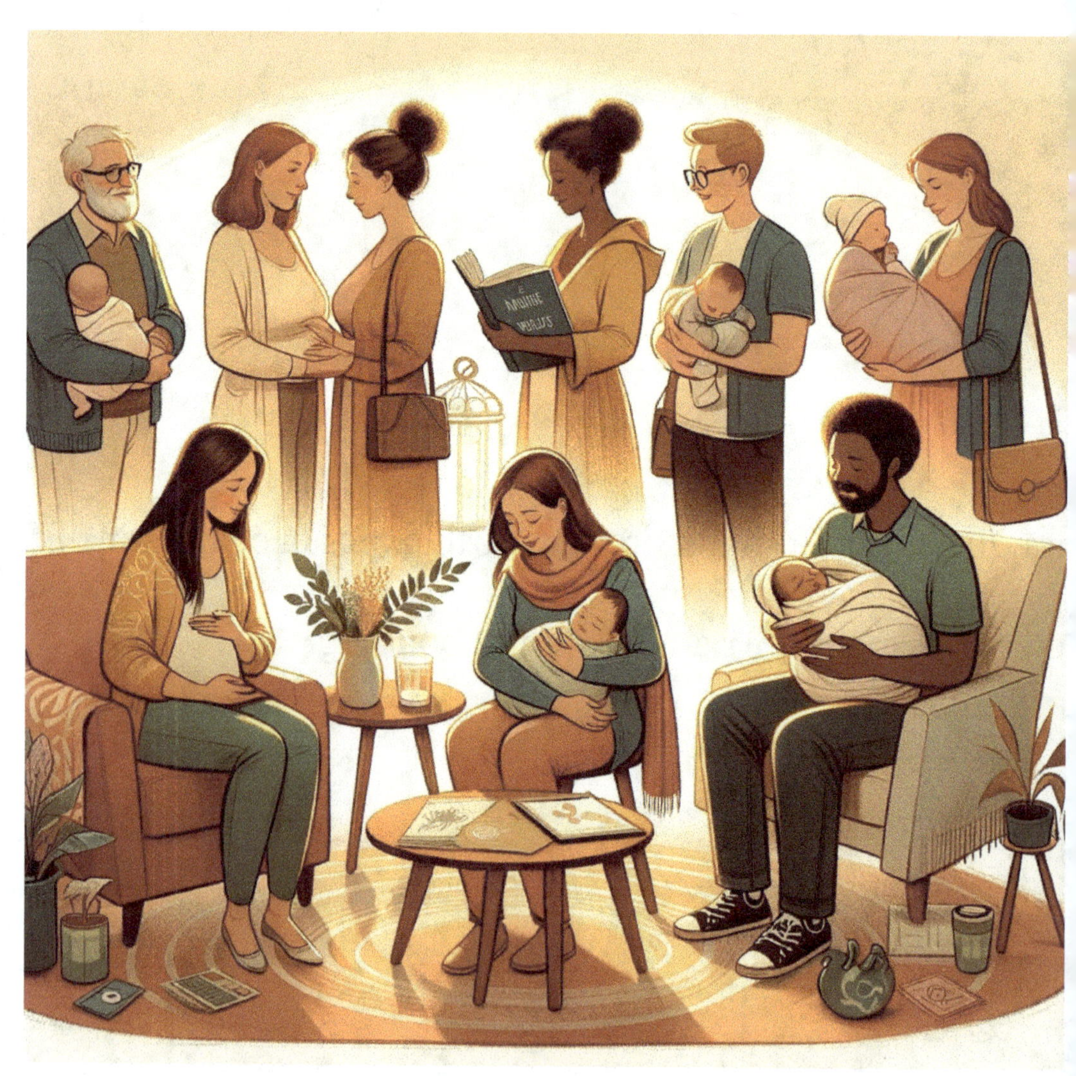

Chapter 4: Choosing the Right Doula

Selecting a doula is a deeply personal decision that can significantly influence your childbirth experience. The right doula not only provides support and knowledge but also aligns with your values, preferences, and personality. This chapter guides you through the process of finding, interviewing, and choosing a doula who is the best fit for your family.

Identifying Your Needs

Reflect on Your Preferences: Begin by considering what kind of birth experience you envision and what role you'd like a doula to play in it. Think about your preferences for communication, support styles (e.g., more hands-on or hands-off), and any specific concerns or fears you have about childbirth.

Consider the Types of Doula Services: As discussed in Chapter 1, there are different types of doulas (birth, postpartum, bereavement, full-spectrum). Determine which type of support you're seeking based on your current needs or situation.

Evaluate Logistical Factors: Availability, location, and cost are practical considerations. Think about your budget for doula services and whether your insurance offers any coverage. Also, consider the doula's availability around your due date and their proximity to your chosen birth location.

Finding and Interviewing Doulas

Where to Look: Start your search by asking for recommendations from friends, family, or your healthcare provider. Online directories, local parenting groups, and social media can also be valuable resources for finding doulas in your area.

Setting Up Interviews: Most doulas offer a free initial consultation or interview. Schedule meetings with several candidates to compare and contrast their personalities, philosophies, and approaches.

Questions to Ask: Prepare a list of questions to ask during the interviews. Consider asking about their training and certification, experience, approach to support, availability for your due date, backup arrangements, and fees. Also, discuss their philosophy on childbirth and postpartum support to ensure it aligns with yours.

Making the Decision

Assessing Compatibility: After the interviews, reflect on which doula you felt most comfortable and connected with. Consider who you believe will best support your needs, preferences, and birth plan.

Consider the Chemistry: The emotional and personal connection is just as important as the doula's qualifications and experience. You should feel comfortable, understood, and respected by your doula.

Check References: Asking for and contacting references can provide additional insights into the doula's practice and the experiences of other families they've supported.

Choosing the right doula is a unique journey for each family, involving careful consideration of personal needs, preferences, and values. By understanding your own needs, thoroughly researching potential doulas, and engaging in open and honest discussions during interviews, you can select a doula who will provide the support, knowledge, and comfort you need during

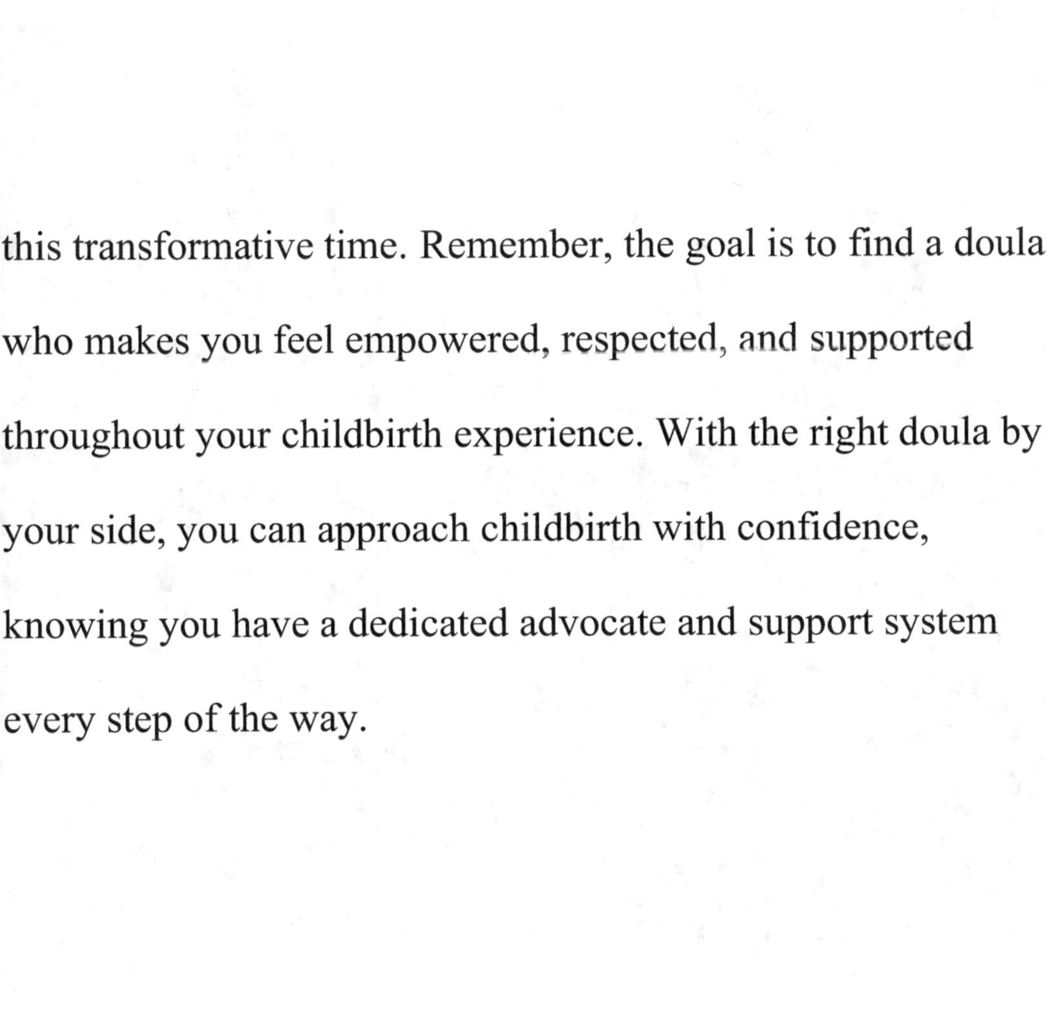

this transformative time. Remember, the goal is to find a doula who makes you feel empowered, respected, and supported throughout your childbirth experience. With the right doula by your side, you can approach childbirth with confidence, knowing you have a dedicated advocate and support system every step of the way.

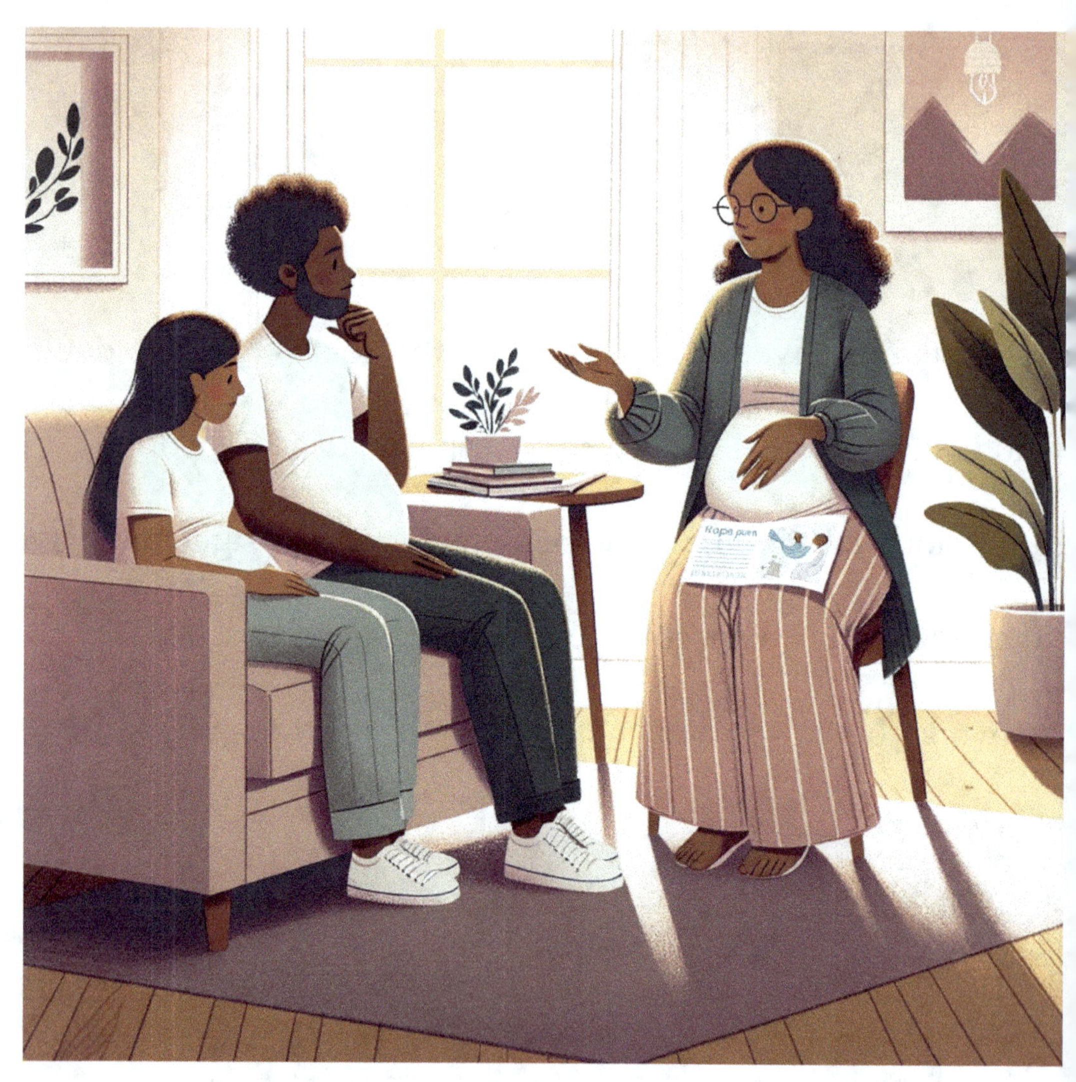

Chapter 5: Working with Your Doula

Once you have chosen a doula, the next steps involve establishing a solid working relationship, setting clear expectations, and understanding how to communicate effectively throughout your journey together. This chapter will guide you through these processes, ensuring that you and your doula are aligned and prepared for the birth and postpartum experience.

Establishing Expectations

Initial Meetings: After hiring your doula, the first step is to have an in-depth meeting (or series of meetings) to discuss your birth plan, fears, preferences, and how you envision your doula supporting you. This is the time to communicate any specific desires, such as how you want to manage pain, the atmosphere you wish to create during labor, and the roles of any other support people present.

Availability and Communication: Clarify expectations around availability, especially as your due date approaches. Discuss how and when to best communicate, whether through phone calls, text messages, or emails, and establish a clear plan for how to reach your doula when you go into labor.

Backup Plans: Talk about backup arrangements in case your doula is unable to attend your birth due to unforeseen circumstances. Meeting the backup doula, if available, can provide peace of mind.

Communication Tips

Open Lines of Communication: Maintain open and honest communication with your doula throughout your pregnancy. Feel free to share updates, concerns, or changes to your birth plan. Your doula is there to support you, and keeping them informed enables them to provide the best possible care.

Feedback Mechanism: Establish a comfortable way to give and receive feedback. If certain support techniques or approaches aren't working for you, it's important to communicate this with your doula so adjustments can be made.

Check-ins: Regular check-ins can help build and maintain a strong relationship with your doula. These can be formal meetings or informal chats to discuss how you're feeling, any new developments, and to revisit your birth plan and expectations as your due date approaches.

Preparing for Birth and Beyond

Birth Plan Review: Work with your doula to review your birth plan, ensuring it reflects your current wishes and includes contingency plans. Your doula can help you consider different scenarios and decisions you might face during labor.

Postpartum Planning: Discuss postpartum support early on. If your doula offers postpartum services, talk about how they can assist with the transition home, breastfeeding support, and newborn care. If your doula does not provide postpartum services, they may be able to recommend resources or other professionals who can help.

Practice and Preparation: Use prenatal visits to practice labor positions, breathing techniques, and other comfort measures. This preparation can help you feel more confident and relaxed as you approach labor and birth.

The relationship you build with your doula is a partnership based on trust, respect, and open communication. By establishing clear expectations, maintaining open lines of communication, and preparing together for birth and the postpartum period, you can create a supportive and empowering environment for your birthing journey. Working with a doula can significantly enhance your experience, providing you with the knowledge, support, and confidence you need to navigate

childbirth and the early days of parenthood.

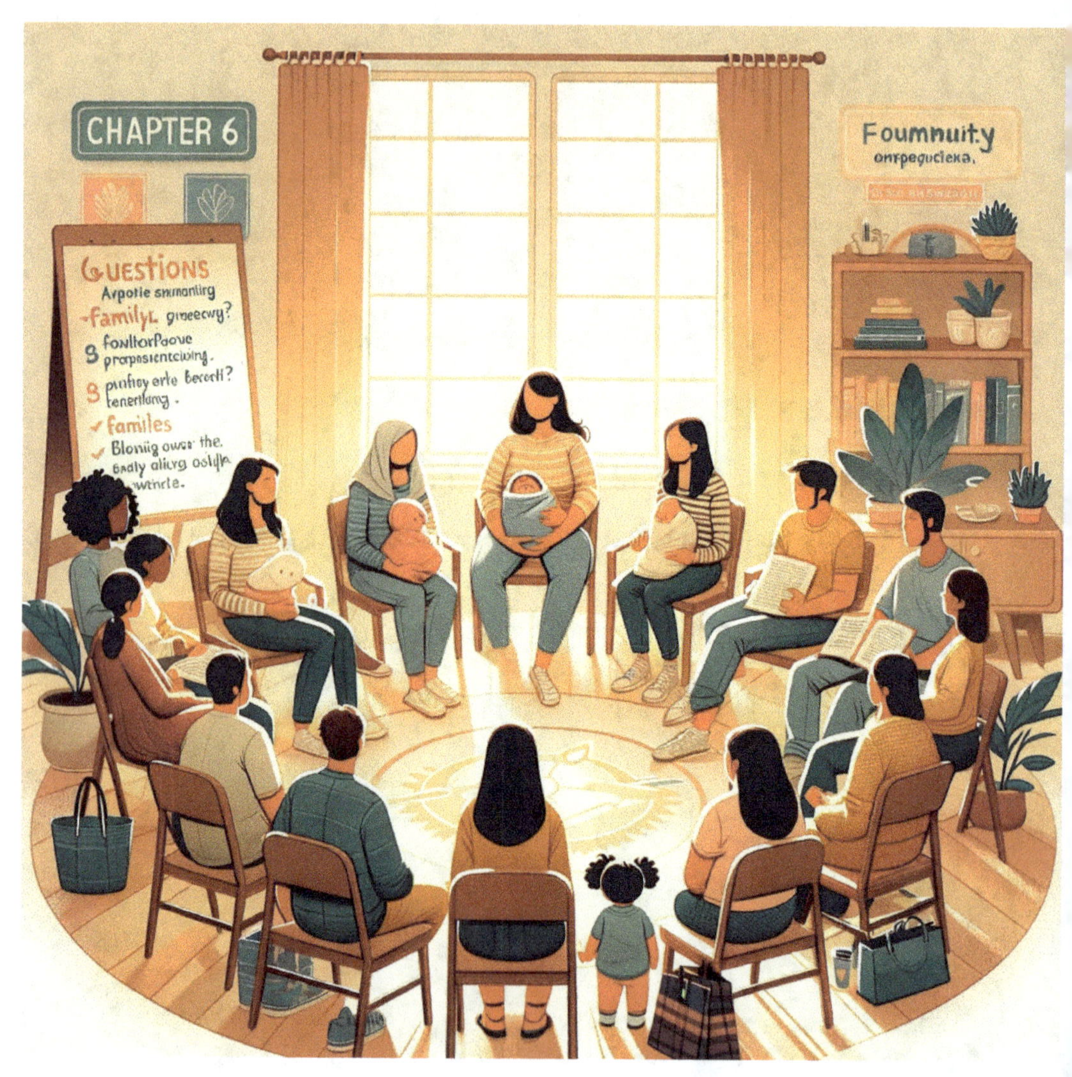

Chapter 6: Frequently Asked Questions

Welcoming a doula into your birthing journey can lead to many questions, especially for families new to the concept of doula care. This chapter addresses some of the most frequently asked questions about doulas, their roles, and how they support families through pregnancy, birth, and the postpartum period.

What exactly does a doula do?

A doula provides continuous emotional, physical, and informational support to the birthing person and their family before, during, and after childbirth. Unlike medical professionals, doulas do not perform clinical tasks but offer support that complements medical care. Their role includes helping the family to understand their options, facilitating communication with healthcare providers, and providing comfort measures and emotional support throughout the childbirth process.

How is a doula different from a midwife?

A midwife is a healthcare professional who provides medical care to pregnant women, delivers babies, and offers postnatal care. Midwives are trained to manage low-risk pregnancies and births, including performing clinical tasks and making medical decisions when necessary. A doula, on the other hand, does not provide medical care but offers support, information, and comfort to the birthing family. Doulas and midwives often work together as part of the birth team, each playing a distinct and complementary role.

Can I have a doula if I plan to give birth in a hospital with an obstetrician?

Yes, you can have a doula regardless of your birth setting or healthcare provider. Doulas support families in hospitals, birth centers, and home births. They work alongside obstetricians, midwives, and nurses, providing continuous support that complements the medical care you receive. It's important to communicate with your healthcare provider about your decision to involve a doula in your birth team so that everyone is aligned with your birth plan and expectations.

Does having a doula reduce the chance of having a cesarean section?

Research suggests that continuous support from a doula is associated with a lower rate of cesarean sections and other interventions. Doulas support the physiological process of childbirth through non-medical means, such as position changes, relaxation techniques, and emotional reassurance, which can contribute to a smoother labor and reduce the need for interventions.

Will a doula make decisions on my behalf?

No, a doula does not make decisions for you. Their role is to provide you with information and support to help you make informed choices about your care. Doulas encourage you to express your preferences and advocate for yourself, ensuring your voice is heard during the birthing process.

Can a doula support my partner too?

Absolutely. Doulas recognize the importance of supporting the entire family, including partners. They can offer guidance on how partners can be involved in the birth process, provide reassurance, and help maintain a calm and supportive environment. This support allows partners to participate in the birth in a way that feels meaningful and supportive to the birthing person.

How much does hiring a doula cost?

The cost of hiring a doula varies depending on their experience, the services offered, and the region. Some doulas offer sliding scale fees, payment plans, or reduced rates for certain circumstances to make their services more accessible. It's worth checking if your health insurance offers any coverage for doula services or if you can use health savings accounts (HSAs) or flexible spending accounts (FSAs) to pay for doula support.

Choosing to include a doula in your birth team is a decision that can significantly enhance your childbirth experience. Doulas provide a unique form of support that complements the medical care you receive, focusing on your emotional, physical, and informational needs throughout the childbirth journey. By understanding the role of a doula and how they can support your family, you can make an informed decision about whether doula care aligns with your needs and preferences for your birth experience.

Appendix A: Resources and References

This appendix serves as a curated collection of resources and references designed to support families in their journey through pregnancy, childbirth, and the postpartum period. Whether seeking more information on doula services, looking for educational material on childbirth, or needing support for breastfeeding, the following resources offer valuable guidance and insight.

Doula Certification Organizations

- **DONA International**

- Website: www.dona.org

- Description: One of the oldest and largest doula certification organizations in the world, offering certification for both birth and postpartum doulas.

- **CAPPA** (Childbirth and Postpartum Professional Association)

- Website: www.cappa.net

- Description: An international certification organization for doulas, childbirth educators, and lactation educators, focusing on a variety of educational programs.

- **Childbirth International** (CBI)

- Website: www.childbirthinternational.com

- Description: Provides training and certification for birth doulas, postpartum doulas, childbirth educators, and breastfeeding counselors worldwide.

Childbirth Education

- **Lamaze International**

  - Website: www.lamaze.org

  - Description: Offers childbirth education classes that promote

a natural, healthy, and safe approach to pregnancy, birth, and

early parenting.

- **The Bradley Method**

  - Website:

www.bradleybirth.com

  - Description: Focuses on natural childbirth and emphasizes the

role of the partner as a birth coach.

- **Evidence Based Birth**

- Website:

www.evidencebasedbirth.com

- Description: An online resource that provides access to research and evidence on various childbirth practices and interventions.

Breastfeeding Support

- **La Leche League International**

  - Website: www.llli.org

  - Description: Offers breastfeeding support, encouragement, information, and education through local meetings and online resources.

- **KellyMom**

  - Website: www.kellymom.com

  - Description: Provides evidence-based information on breastfeeding, sleep, and parenting.

- **International Lactation Consultant Association** (ILCA)

  - Website: www.ilca.org

  - Description: Find a lactation consultant near you to get

professional breastfeeding support and advice.

Parenting and Postpartum Support

- **Postpartum Support International** (PSI)

  - Website: www.postpartum.net

  - Description: Offers support to families experiencing

postpartum depression, anxiety, and other mood disorders,

including a helpline and local support groups.

- **The Bump**

- Website: www.thebump.com

- Description: A comprehensive resource for all things pregnancy and baby, offering articles, tools, and a supportive community.

- **What to Expect**

- Website: www.whattoexpect.com

- Description: Provides a wealth of information on pregnancy, childbirth, and the first years of parenting, based on the best-selling book series.

Online Communities

- **BabyCenter Community**

- Website: community.babycenter.com

- Description: An online forum where parents and parents-to-be can discuss pregnancy, babies, and toddlers with peers.

- **Mothering Forums**

  - Website: www.mothering.com/community

  - **Description**: A supportive community for parents focused on natural living and attachment parenting.

These resources represent just a fraction of the vast amount of information available to families. By exploring these websites and organizations, you can deepen your understanding of childbirth, enhance your preparation for parenting, and find supportive communities to join on your journey.

Appendix B: Glossary

This glossary provides definitions for terms related to doula care, childbirth, and the postpartum period. Understanding these terms can help families navigate the wealth of information available and make informed decisions about their care.

- **Birth Doula**: A trained professional who provides continuous physical, emotional, and informational support to a birthing person before, during, and shortly after childbirth to help them achieve the healthiest, most satisfying experience possible.

- **Postpartum Doula**: A trained professional who provides emotional, physical, and informational support to a family after the birth of a baby, helping them to adjust to the new family dynamics, offering care tips for the newborn, and providing assistance with feeding and household organization.

- **Bereavement Doula**: A trained professional who provides support to families experiencing a loss during pregnancy or after childbirth, including miscarriage, stillbirth, or neonatal death. This support can include emotional, physical, and informational assistance as families navigate their grief.

- **Full-Spectrum Doula**: A doula who offers a wide range of services, supporting individuals and families through various reproductive experiences, including birth, postpartum, miscarriage, abortion, and fertility challenges.

- **Effacement:** The process by which the cervix becomes thinner and softer in preparation for childbirth. It is measured as a percentage, from 0% (no effacement) to 100% (fully effaced).

- **Dilation**: The widening of the cervix measured in centimeters, from 0 (closed) to 10 (fully dilated), indicating readiness for childbirth.

- **Engagement**: Refers to the baby descending into the pelvis, indicating the beginning of the labor process. Also known as "dropping" or "lightening."

- **Epidural**: A common form of pain relief used during labor, administered via an injection into the epidural space of the spine, which blocks nerve signals from the lower part of the body.

- **Pitocin**: A synthetic form of oxytocin used to induce or augment labor. It can be administered intravenously to stimulate uterine contractions.

- **Water Birth**: A birthing process in which the birthing person labors and/or delivers in a tub of warm water, which can help to manage pain and facilitate a more gentle birth.

- **Skin-to-Skin Contact**: The practice of placing the newborn directly on the birthing person's chest immediately after birth, which promotes bonding and has been shown to have numerous health benefits for both the baby and the parent.

- **Lactation Consultant**: A healthcare professional specialized in breastfeeding support, including addressing breastfeeding challenges, offering advice on feeding positions, and providing information on milk production.

- **Placenta Encapsulation**: The process of dehydrating the placenta, grinding it into a powder, and encapsulating it into pills for the birthing person to consume postpartum. Some believe it can help in the recovery process, though scientific evidence supporting these claims is limited.

- **Lochia**: The vaginal discharge following childbirth, containing blood, mucus, and uterine tissue. It typically lasts for several weeks as the body heals and returns to its pre-pregnancy state.

This glossary is designed to familiarize readers with common terms they may encounter during their journey through pregnancy, childbirth, and the postpartum period.

Appendix C: Interview Questions for Potential Doulas

Selecting a doula is a significant decision that can greatly influence your childbirth experience. To assist you in finding a doula who aligns with your needs and preferences, consider asking the following questions during your interviews. These questions are designed to help you understand the doula's experience, approach, and compatibility with your family.

General Background and Experience

1. Can you tell us about your training and certifications? Are you affiliated with any doula organizations?

2. How long have you been working as a doula, and how many families have you supported?

3. What inspired you to become a doula?

Approach to Doula Support

4. How would you describe your philosophy on childbirth and supporting families during the birth process?

5. Can you walk us through how you typically support families before, during, and after birth?

6. How do you tailor your support to meet the diverse needs and preferences of different families?

Availability and Logistics

7. Are you available around my estimated due date?

8. What is your policy on backup doulas? Can we meet them in advance?

9. How do you handle communication with clients? What is your response time to calls or messages?

Support During Labor and Birth

10. How do you support the birthing person and their partner during labor and delivery?

11. Can you provide examples of pain management and comfort measures you recommend or assist with?

12. How do you work alongside healthcare providers in a hospital, birth center, or home birth setting?

Postpartum Support

13. Do you offer postpartum support? If so, what does that include?

14. How do you support breastfeeding and addressing any challenges that may arise?

15. Can you provide resources or referrals for additional postpartum services, such as lactation consultants or mental health professionals?

Fees and Contractual Details

16. What are your fees, and what services do they include?

17. Do you offer any packages or additional services?

18. Can you explain your contract terms, including payment plans, refund policies, and what happens in the event you cannot attend the birth?

Compatibility and Communication

19. How do you ensure clear and effective communication with the families you support?

20. In what ways do you support the partner's involvement in the birth process?

21. How do you handle situations where medical interventions are proposed or required during labor and birth?

22. Is there anything else we should know about you or your approach to doula support?

23. Can you provide references from families you've supported in the past?

These questions are a starting point for your conversations with potential doulas. Feel free to add, modify, or skip questions based on your specific concerns and priorities. The most important outcome is that you feel confident and comfortable with the doula you choose to support your family during this transformative time.

Appendix D: Birth Plan Template

Creating a birth plan is a valuable exercise for expectant parents to articulate their preferences for the birth experience and communicate these wishes to their healthcare team. This template is designed to guide you through considering various aspects of labor, delivery, and postpartum care. Remember, flexibility is key, as birth can be unpredictable. Use this template as a starting point to discuss options with your doula and healthcare provider.

Personal Information

- **Name**:

- **Partner's Name** (if applicable):

- **Due Date**:

- **Healthcare Provider**:

- **Birth Location**:

Labor Preferences

- **People Present During Labor**: (List who you would like to have in the room, including family, friends, doula, etc.)

- **Environment**: (Preferences for lighting, music, bringing personal items, etc.)

- **Mobility:** (Preferences about walking, changing positions, use of birthing ball, etc.)

- **Monitoring**: (Preferences for fetal heart rate monitoring - continuous vs. intermittent)

- **Pain Management**: (Natural techniques you wish to try, circumstances under which you would consider medication, specific medications you prefer or wish to avoid)

- **Hydration and Nutrition**: (Preferences regarding eating and drinking during labor)

Delivery Preferences

- **Position for Delivery**: (Upright, squatting, on back, etc.)

- **Use of Mirrors**: (To watch the birth, if desired)

- **Touching the Head**: (Preference to feel the baby's head as it crowns)

- **Assisted Delivery**: (Thoughts on the use of forceps or vacuum extraction)

- **Episiotomy**: (Conditions under which you would or would not want one)

Immediately After Birth

- **Skin-to-Skin Contact**: (Your wishes regarding immediate skin-to-skin contact with your baby)

- **Umbilical Cord Cutting**: (Who you would like to cut the cord and timing - immediate or delayed clamping)

- **Placenta Delivery**: (Natural delivery of the placenta or use of medication to assist)

- **Use of Synthetic Oxytocin Post Delivery**: (Preferences regarding its use after delivery to contract the uterus)

Newborn Care Preferences

- **Initial Medical Assessments**: (In-room with you, preferences if baby needs to be taken to NICU)

- **Feeding**: (Breastfeeding immediately, use of formula, etc.)

- **Bathing**: (Timing of the first bath)

- **Vitamin K, Hepatitis B Vaccination, and Eye Ointment**:
(Preferences for these newborn procedures)

In Case of Cesarean

- **Presence of Partner/Doula**: (Who you would like to
accompany you if possible)

- **Anesthesia Preferences**: (If any specific preferences exist)

- **Skin-to-Skin Contact After C-Section**: (When and how you
would like this to occur)

- **Recovery**: (Preferences regarding recovery room and initial
breastfeeding support)

Postpartum Care

- **Rooming-In**: (Whether you want your baby to stay in the room with you at all times)

- **Visitors**: (Preferences regarding visitors in the hospital)

- **Feeding**: (Breastfeeding support, formula feeding preferences)

- **Discharge Education**: (Specific topics you would like information on before going home)

This birth plan template is a tool to help you think about and communicate your preferences. However, it's important to discuss each item with your healthcare provider and doula to understand the options and potential need for flexibility based on how labor and delivery unfold.

Appendix E: Postpartum Plan Template

The transition to life with a new baby is a significant change that can be both joyous and challenging. Creating a postpartum plan can help you anticipate your needs and set up a support system in advance. This template covers various aspects of postpartum life, from self-care for the birthing person to infant care and household management. Use this template as a guide to discuss and plan with your partner, family, and support network.

Personal Information

- **Name**:

- **Partner's Name** (if applicable):

- **Baby's Due Date/Birth Date**:

- **Contact Information for Healthcare Providers**:

(Pediatrician, Obstetrician, Midwife, Lactation Consultant)

Recovery and Self-Care

Physical Recovery:

- Care for perineal area or cesarean incision

- Pain management plan

- Follow-up medical appointments

Emotional Well-being:

- Signs of postpartum mood disorders to watch for

- Support resources (therapist, support groups, hotlines)

- Strategies for managing emotional highs and lows

Nutrition:

- Meal planning and preparation (consider meal train, freezer meals)

- Hydration goals

- Supplements or vitamins

Rest and Sleep:

- Sleep strategy for the birthing person

- Sharing nighttime responsibilities

Baby Care

Feeding:

- Breastfeeding plan and support

- Formula feeding plan (if applicable)

- Feeding schedule or cues to watch for

Sleep:

- Baby sleep area setup

- Sleep safety practices

- Approach to nighttime awakenings

Healthcare:

- Schedule for pediatric appointments

- Vaccination plan

- Tracking baby's growth and milestones

Household Management

Chores and Responsibilities:

- Division of household tasks

- Hiring professional help (cleaning service, postpartum doula)

- Grocery shopping and errands plan

Sibling and Pet Care:

- Adjustments for older siblings

- Plan for introducing baby to pets

- Childcare arrangements for siblings

Support System

Visitors:

- Guidelines for visitors in the early weeks

- Support tasks visitors can help with

Professional Support:

- List of postpartum professionals (doula, lactation consultant, therapist)

- Community resources and support groups

Partner/Co-Parent Support:

- Communication plan for sharing feelings and needs

- Date nights or couple time

Special Considerations

Returning to Work:

- Maternity/paternity leave duration

- Childcare plans

- Transition plan for returning to work

Physical Activity and Hobbies:

- Plan for resuming exercise or hobbies

- Activities for relaxation and self-care

Additional Notes:

This postpartum plan template is a starting point for preparing for the weeks and months after your baby's arrival. Discussing and filling out this plan with your support network can help ensure that you have the help and resources you need during this significant transition period.

Conclusion

As we reach the conclusion of "What is a Doula? The Guidebook for Every Family," it's important to reflect on the journey we've embarked upon together. From understanding the pivotal role of doulas in childbirth and postpartum care to navigating the process of choosing and working with a doula, our goal has been to demystify this invaluable support system and highlight its benefits for families of all kinds.

Doulas, with their compassionate presence and expert guidance, offer more than just support during labor and delivery. They empower families, advocate for the birthing person's wishes, and facilitate a positive and transformative birth experience. The evidence is clear: the presence of a doula can significantly improve birth outcomes, reduce the need for interventions, and enhance the emotional well-being of the entire family.

Choosing to include a doula in your birth team is a deeply personal decision—one that can shape your birth experience in profound ways. As we've explored in this guidebook, the right doula can offer not only comfort and support but also a wealth of knowledge and advocacy, ensuring that your voice is heard and respected throughout the childbirth process.

However, the journey doesn't end with the birth of your child. The postpartum period is a critical time of adjustment and growth for new families. Here, too, doulas play a crucial role, offering guidance, support, and resources to navigate the challenges and joys of early parenthood. Whether through direct postpartum support or by connecting families with additional resources, doulas help to lay the foundation for a healthy and happy start to life with your new addition.

In writing this guidebook, we've aimed to provide a comprehensive resource for families considering doula support. We hope that the information, insights, and personal stories shared within these pages have illuminated the path for those curious about what a doula can bring to their birth experience.

Remember, every family's journey is unique, and the decision to work with a doula is as individual as the families themselves.

As you move forward, whether you're anticipating the arrival of a new family member or supporting someone who is, may this guidebook serve as a beacon of knowledge and empowerment. The birth of a child is one of life's most extraordinary events, and with the right support, it can be an experience filled with joy, respect, and profound connection.

Thank you for allowing us to be part of your journey to understanding the vital role of doulas in childbirth and beyond. May your path forward be enriched by the support, wisdom, and care that a doula can provide, making your birth experience as positive and empowering as possible.

Wishing you a beautiful birthing journey and a joyful beginning to life with your new baby.

* 9 7 9 8 8 8 4 8 0 8 6 1 4 *